Daniela Santana Portes

Access to medicines:

Daniela Santana Portes

Access to medicines:

A study based on the perceptions of users of Basic Health Units in Divinópolis, Minas Gerais

ScienciaScripts

Imprint
Any brand names and product names mentioned in this book are subject to trademark, brand or patent protection and are trademarks or registered trademarks of their respective holders. The use of brand names, product names, common names, trade names, product descriptions etc. even without a particular marking in this work is in no way to be construed to mean that such names may be regarded as unrestricted in respect of trademark and brand protection legislation and could thus be used by anyone.

Cover image: www.ingimage.com

This book is a translation from the original published under ISBN 978-613-9-64734-7.

Publisher:
Sciencia Scripts
is a trademark of
Dodo Books Indian Ocean Ltd. and OmniScriptum S.R.L publishing group

120 High Road, East Finchley, London, N2 9ED, United Kingdom
Str. Armeneasca 28/1, office 1, Chisinau MD-2012, Republic of Moldova, Europe
Printed at: see last page
ISBN: 978-620-7-77886-7

ACKNOWLEDGEMENTS

After completing what is considered an important stage, I must thank everyone involved, who directly or indirectly contributed to my being able to finish my degree and become a professional.

To God, who out of his infinite goodness sustained me so that I could walk my dreamed-of paths, who gave me the gift of learning and placed in me an infinite desire to contribute to the good of my neighbour. By your grace, I realise that when we research, understand and succeed, we are clearly getting closer to you and your work.

Huge gratitude to my parents, who have always made my dreams their goals. For teaching me the value of knowledge and fighting so that I could embrace the opportunities they didn't have. For being my first and eternal mentors, giving meaning to the word education in the most loving way possible. Thank you for lovingly shaping my personal and professional being!

To my grandparents for their intense prayers and understanding during my many moments of absence. In particular, to my grandmother Luzia for being the first patient with whom I practised Pharmaceutical Care and for always listening to my advice regarding the use of medicines, even without following it. It was by trying to pass on some of what I was learning that I learnt a lot about respecting the patient's beliefs and subjective experiences.

I couldn't fail to thank my aunt Luciana, who was an example of determination and dedication to her studies. Initially, you served as a source of inspiration in my professional career and I confess that it was a challenge for me to get rid of your image. Today I see with total clarity that although we chose the same profession, we have visions and experiences that add up, but above all make us different professionals, each with their own way of promoting health.

To my uncle Edson for watching me grow up and praying for me to grow up in grace and wisdom. I hope that your wishes have been granted and that, in a way, you are proud to have been part of my growth in such an intense and loving way. To my uncle Wanderson for believing in me even when I had the terrible habit of minimising my own achievements. After our conversations, which were always very enlightening and encouraging, the world always opened up to me and that's how I began to believe more in my potential.

I would especially like to thank my boyfriend, Diego, for being by my side from when this whole path was still glimpsed with many uncertainties. For supporting all my decisions, sharing all the details of graduating and writing this work. For being a motivator and for learning with me to advise and to silence, to support and also to criticise when necessary. For being a comforting shoulder when I needed one, even when I couldn't reciprocate. Thank you for dreaming with me and for being part of each other's goals.

To my colleagues in Pharmacy 140 for taking on the challenge of unveiling the new together. To my colleagues in the Hospital Pharmacy and Health Services programme for sharing the same ideals.

It is essential to thank the friends I made during my degree for being constant gifts on my journey. Especially Amana and Amanda for always being there for me, especially recently, sharing worries, anxieties, joys and, above all, smiles every day. Thank you for your constant complicity, girls!

I would also like to thank my final internship mates Marina Dias, Marina Alves and Caludiane for patiently listening to my comments on this work and sharing their experiences with me.

My gratitude for the internship, monitoring, IC and project opportunities I had during my degree, represented by the ICB Monitoring Department, UFMG Hospital das Clínicas, PNAUM and João XXIII Hospital.

To the René Rachou Research Centre - Fiocruz Minas, especially the Transdisciplinary Studies Group in Education, Health and the Environment

(GETESA) for the knowledge I was able to acquire during my time as a Scientific Initiate and for the structure to carry out this work To the Servir Project team, especially my co-supervisor Dr Tatiana Chama for the opportunity as a scholarship holder in the Project and for the unique guidance provided during the construction of this work.

To Professor Maria Auxiliadora Martins for accepting the guidance of this work and collaborating in making it possible to complete it.

My eternal gratitude goes to all the undergraduate teachers who passed on their knowledge and experience and were true encouragers in building professionals committed to science and the well-being of the population.

To the Federal University of Minas Gerais and the Faculty of Pharmacy for being favourable environments for the transmission of knowledge and the training of professionals who are aware of and committed to social needs.

To FUMP for their assistance during the course, providing subsidies so that I could devote myself to my studies without too many worries.

Finally, I'll end by making it clear that any and all words written here will never be enough or succeed in expressing my real gratitude to everyone involved in this stage and throughout my undergraduate career. In any case, I leave you with this way of expressing my thanks and with the expectation that taking new paths will increasingly reaffirm the importance of all of you, right from the start.

SUMMARY

Pharmaceutical services are part of Pharmaceutical Assistance, are part of health services and aim to guarantee qualified access to medicines for the population in a comprehensive and continuous manner. In Primary Health Care, the minimum structuring of these services, as well as user guidance activities, is recommended in the Guidelines and Manuals of Brazilian health organisations. However, studies have shown various organisational and structural problems in these services, which compromise guaranteed access to medicines. Considering the difficulties faced by users in obtaining their medicines with the proper guidance, this study aimed to find out the perceptions of users of pharmaceutical services in the Basic Health Units of Divinópolis, Minas Gerais, in relation to access to medicines. The research was based on the Servir Project, a qualitative study carried out in 2014. Data related to the sociodemographic, economic and health profile of users, perceptions about the physical structure of the services, obtaining medicines and dispensing practices were extracted from the Servir Project database. The data was categorised, a new database was created and the data was quantified. Sixty-nine users took part in the investigation and according to the users' perceptions, three dimensions of the concept of access (WHO, 2000) were identified: availability, adequacy and quality of services. In the physical availability dimension, it was observed that only 47.8 per cent of users were able to obtain all the medicines prescribed. In terms of adequacy, the majority of interviewees rated the physical space, comfort of the pharmacy dispensing areas and waiting times as inadequate. The quality of the services offered was considered unsatisfactory in terms of providing basic information to users of medicines in the services studied. It is therefore necessary to implement improvements aimed at local Pharmaceutical Services in order to guarantee qualified access to medicines for the population.

Keywords: Access. Medicines. Pharmaceutical services. Primary Health

Care.

SUMMARY

CHAPTER 1

INTRODUCTION

Primary Health Care (PHC) is considered the preferred contact for users and the main gateway to Brazil's Unified Health System (SUS). In this context, Pharmaceutical Services (PS) plays an important role in health care, as it seeks to guarantee access and promote the rational use of medicines, aimed at meeting the therapeutic needs of the population, with sufficiency, regularity and appropriate quality, in order to provide guidance for the rational use of medicines, as proposed in the National Pharmaceutical Services Policy (BRASIL, 2004; BRASIL, 2014).

Pharmaceutical services are part of PS and are included in health services. Particularly in PHC, these services seek to guarantee comprehensive and continuous care for the health needs and problems of the population, both individual and collective, with medicines as one of the essential elements, contributing to their equitable access and rational use (PAHO, 2013).

In order to achieve these objectives, pharmaceutical services in PHC must have a minimum structure that allows them to carry out their activities (BRASIL, 2016), such as an adequate physical area and equipment, as well as trained human resources to carry out all the activities that this service is responsible for, such as applying knowledge about medicines and therapy, as well as communication skills, in order to establish a relationship with service users and the team of health professionals (BRASIL, 2009).

Despite the existence of Pharmaceutical Services with recognised pharmaceutical services, consolidated and structured by provisions such as Laws, Ordinances and other official documents such as guides, reports and manuals (BRASIL, 1998; 2006b; 2007; 2009; 2014), the reality shows various organisational and structural problems in these places. In general, actions are centred on technical-managerial activities focused on the medicine and not on the user (PEREIRA *et al.,* 2015) and various deficiencies persist, ranging from inadequate infrastructure to the unavailability of medicines in Brazilian pharmaceutical services (GUERRA *et a!,* 2004; VIEIRA, 2008; MENDES *et al.,* 2014; PANIZ et *al.,* 2016).

Considering the difficulties faced by users in obtaining their medicines from PHC pharmaceutical services, an investigation was carried out, the Servir Project: evaluation of the role of pharmaceutical services in access to medicines in Divinópolis, Minas Gerais, by the Transdisciplinary Health Education and Environment Studies Group of the René Rachou Research Centre (GETESA/CPqRR/Fiocruz) (LUZ *et al.,* 2013). The main objective of the Servir Project was to assess the role of pharmaceutical services in providing access to medicines in a medium-sized municipality, in this case the municipality of Divinópolis, according to the perceptions of managers, health professionals and users.

This study is part of the Servir Project and aimed to find out about users' perceptions of access to medicines in these pharmaceutical services in Divinópolis, Minas Gerais.

CHAPTER 2

LITERATURE REVIEW

2.1 Pharmaceutical Services in Primary Health Care

Pharmaceutical Assistance began with the creation of the Central de Medicamentos (CEME) in 1971, and was thus established as a public policy. The CEME was set up with the aim of improving access to medicines, especially for the population with lower purchasing power, and its mission was to supply medicines to the low income population. It also aimed to promote and organise pharmaceutical assistance activities for this population, with a centralised policy for the acquisition and distribution of medicines in the country (BRASIL, 1971; OLIVEIRA *etaL,* 2010).

In order to improve the supply of medicines to the states, the Basic Pharmacy was set up in 1987 with the aim of rationalising the availability of medicines for PHC. The Basic Pharmacy was idealised as a standard module of medicines selected from the National List of Medicines (RENAME) that allowed for the treatment of the most common diseases of the Brazilian population. The modules contained 48 medicines and were designed to meet the needs of 3,000 people over a six-month period. However, although the implementation of the Basic Pharmacy took regional diversities into account, the centralisation of the programming and procurement processes did not take these diversities into account, since the same standard module was supplied to all regions of Brazil, and was therefore abolished in 1988 (COSENDEY, 2000).

In 1997, still under the management of the CEME, the Basic Pharmacy Programme (PFB) was created to meet the need for basic medicines and was the first pharmaceutical care initiative to focus on PHC. The selection of medicines was based mainly on CEME's previous experience and the pharmaceutical assistance programmes of the states of Paraná, São Paulo and Minas Gerais. Thus, the PFB was developed along the same lines as the Basic Pharmacy, but distribution control was decentralised and the hubs were coordinated by official producer laboratories that sent the medicines to the municipalities via the Brazilian Post and Telegraph Company. This process made deliveries quicker and gave greater control over distribution (BRASIL, 1997; COSENDEY, 2000).

During the CEME's existence, several problems were detected in relation to the population's access to medicines, including wastage of medicines due mainly to poor knowledge of the epidemiological profile of the populations served, logistical difficulties resulting in large losses of medicines and insufficient financial resources (ACURCIO, 2003). Then, in August 1997, due to a series of political frictions and corruption scandals, the CEME was abolished and its activities were distributed between different bodies within the Ministry of Health and the PFB was now coordinated by the Ministry of Health's Directorate of Strategic Programmes (COSENDEY, 2000; OLIVEIRA *et al.,* 2010).

Also noteworthy was the regulation of the Unified Health System through Law No. 8.080/90, known as the Organic Health Law, which defined the formulation of a medicines policy and included the "execution of comprehensive therapeutic assistance actions, including pharmaceutical assistance" (BRASIL, 1990). This context further reinforced the need to formulate a national medicines policy in line with the regulations of the country's new health system (OLIVEIRA *et al.,* 2010).

In 1998, the PFB was reformulated and no longer had the participation of the state level. This led the programme in the opposite direction to the process of organising and decentralising Pharmaceutical Services that was beginning in several states. It also failed to meet the need for the PFB to interact with and adapt to these initiatives (COSENDEY, 2000).

Given this scenario, the National Medicines Policy (PNM) was drawn up and published in 1998, with the aim of "guaranteeing the necessary safety, efficacy and quality of medicines, promoting their rational use and giving the population access to those considered essential" (BRASIL, 1998). The basic premise is the decentralisation of the acquisition and distribution of essential medicines, respecting the needs of local populations through epidemiological criteria, and from then on the process of decentralising pharmaceutical assistance in the SUS began.

The PNM defined Pharmaceutical Assistance as:

> Group of activities related to medicines, aimed at supporting the health actions demanded by a community. It involves the supply of medicines in each and every one of their constituent stages, conservation and quality control, the safety and therapeutic efficacy of medicines, the monitoring and evaluation of their use, obtaining and disseminating information about medicines and the ongoing education of health professionals, patients and the community to ensure the rational use of medicines (BRASIL, 1998. p. 13).

Marin *et al.* (2003) also clarify that, for Brazil, the term Pharmaceutical Services involves comprehensive, multi-professional and intersectoral activities whose object of work is the organisation of actions and services related to medicines in their various dimensions, but mainly with an emphasis on the relationship with the patient and the community with a view to promoting health. In 2004, the National Health Council published the National Pharmaceutical Assistance Policy (PNAF), which reinforces the idea that pharmaceutical assistance is part of individual or collective health care, with medicines as an essential input, access to which must be guaranteed along with rational use (BRASIL, 2004).

The various debates on the reorientation of pharmaceutical services, the publication of the PNM and the divergence of the Basic Pharmacy Programme from the needs of the Brazilian population led to the programme being discontinued in its current form. So, in line with the process of decentralising the SUS and Pharmaceutical Services, in 1999 GM/MS Ordinance No. 176 was published, establishing the IAFB (Incentive for Basic Pharmaceutical

Services) (BRASIL, 1999; VIEIRA, 2010).

The IAFB established a series of criteria for qualifying municipalities and states for Basic Pharmaceutical Assistance and defined the amounts to be transferred for the purchase of essential medicines (BRASIL, 1999). Unlike the Basic Pharmacy Programme, the IAFB covered all municipalities and began to count on the participation of state and municipal managers in the acquisition and distribution of medicines, involving these spheres in the process of managing Pharmaceutical Services (BRASIL, 2007). This incentive aimed to increase the population's access to medicines and was the initial step towards decentralising pharmaceutical services (BRASIL, 2001).

In 2007, the Ministry of Health reorganised the federal funding of Pharmaceutical Assistance, which is intended for the acquisition of medicines to be offered to the population, especially in SUS outpatient services. In this way, programmes were grouped into components, one of which was the Basic Component of Pharmaceutical Assistance (BRASIL, 2007).

The Basic Component of Pharmaceutical Assistance is intended for the acquisition of medicines and pharmaceutical supplies, including those related to specific health problems and programmes, within the scope of Primary Health Care, i.e. highly prevalent diseases that affect the population and require low-tech care. The list of medicines is selected to address the majority of the population's health problems, although it can be supplemented with other medicines from standardised lists, such as the current State List of Essential Medicines (RESME) and Municipal List of Essential Medicines (REMUNE), defined according to the epidemiological profile of each state and/or municipality (BRASIL, 2013).

Its implementation is decentralised, with municipalities, the Federal District and the states being responsible for organising pharmaceutical services in accordance with their respective defined activities, including the selection, programming, acquisition, storage (including stock control and expiry dates for medicines), distribution and dispensing of the medicines and supplies for which they are responsible. Medicines are dispensed in the pharmacies of basic health units, under the responsibility of the municipal health departments and on presentation of a medical prescription (BRASIL, 2013).

2.2 Pharmaceutical Services

According to Zuluaga (2013), in Brazil, the use of the term Pharmaceutical Services (PS) is still being consolidated and because it is a recent conceptualisation in the country, there is confusion about the terminology and concept in the literature.

Historically, the term comes from the literal translation of *pharmaceutical services in* English or *servidos farmacêuticos in* Spanish and, according to the Health Sciences descriptors of the Virtual Health Library, it is the Spanish descriptor for Pharmaceutical *Services.* However, in Brazil, the term Pharmaceutical Services has gained greater coverage and has been adopted, but with its own contours and meanings. Thus, different concepts of PS and FS are used in Brazil, with Pharmaceutical Services involving aspects such as research, development and production of drugs, as discussed above, while the term Pharmaceutical Services involves activities more related to health units and is understood as a set of actions contained in PS (PINHEIRO, 2010; PEREIRA et *al.,* 2015).

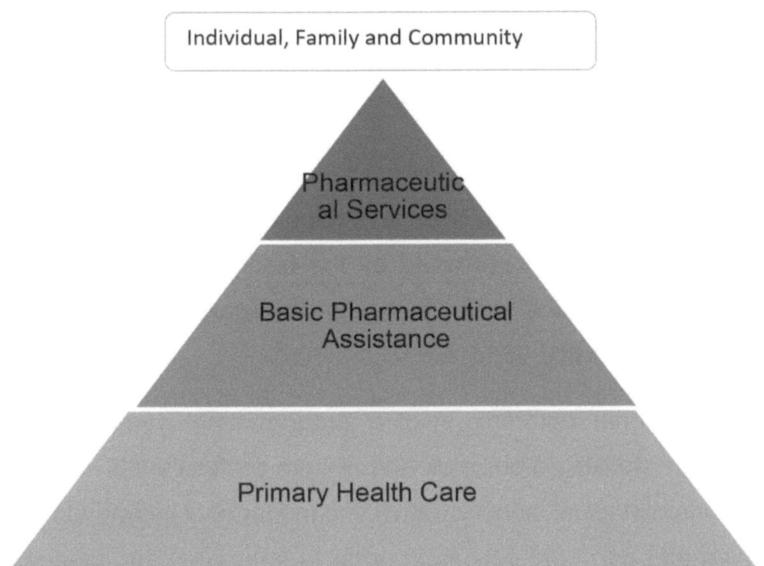

Figure 1. Organisation of Pharmaceutical Services in Primary Health Care

Source: Adapted from Pereira, 2013.

In Figure 1, you can better understand the difference between the terms and see that Pharmaceutical Services are part of health services and are closely linked to PS from the first level of care and seek to ensure that the population's needs are met, both individually and collectively (PAHO, 2013).

According to the document *Pharmaceutical Services based on Primary Health Care* (PAHO, 2013), Pharmaceutical Services based on Primary Health Care are defined as:

> A set of actions in the health system that seek to guarantee comprehensive, integrated and continuous care for the health needs and problems of the population, both individual and collective, with medicines as one of the essential elements, contributing to their equitable access and rational use. These actions should be carried out by pharmacists or under their coordination, incorporated into the health team with a view to improving the population's quality of life (PAHO, 2013, p. 3).

The purpose of Pharmaceutical Services activities is to provide qualified access to essential medicines made available by the public network and their actions are fundamental in achieving the objectives of treatment, such as re-establishing health conditions in the shortest possible time, with the least occurrence of harm to the patient and at the lowest cost to the health system (PAHO, 2013; ZULUAGA, 2013).

In Brazil, Pharmaceutical Services in PHC, as a component of health actions, must comply with the guidelines proposed by the National Pharmaceutical Services Policy and represent a set of technical-managerial and technical-assistance procedures (BRASIL, 2014; BRASIL, 2009).

Technical and managerial activities involve programming, requisitioning, storing, receiving and stocking medicines and require professionals who are trained to apply epidemiological, administrative and managerial knowledge and information to plan and carry out actions in order to guarantee the adequate availability of medicines, with good quality and conservation.

The development of technical-assistance activities includes the dispensing process, as well as pharmaceutical guidance and pharmacotherapeutic follow-up of patients, and requires teams trained to apply knowledge about medicines, therapeutics, as well as skills, especially in communication, to establish relationships with service users and the team of health professionals, with the aim of guaranteeing the effectiveness and safety of treatments and enabling the evaluation of results. Other activities included in the pharmacist's assistance activities are health education and technical support by the pharmacist for the health team, in order to disseminate information about medicines and health to the population and the team (PAHO, 2013; BRAZIL, 2009).

With regard to the minimum structure for the proper execution of pharmaceutical services, it is important to emphasise the need for a physical area, equipment and trained human resources to carry out all the activities that this service is responsible for. Marin *et al.* (2003) also point out that it is essential to draw up technical norms, standard operating procedures and control instruments to record all the information relating to the work processes carried out.

Despite the legal orientation in Brazil for PS and FS to be recognised, consolidated and structured, there are many organisational, financial and infrastructure problems that point to the fragility and poor quality of the services in operation in the country.

According to data from the Systematic Survey of Service Research and Household Research on Access to Medicines (PDAUM), carried out in Brazil in 2004, the average availability for the main medicines was 74% in public health units (PAHO, 2005). A study carried out with data from 38,812 Brazilian Basic Health Units (UBS) found that the average availability of medicines was 56 per cent (MENDES *et al*, 2014). Guerra *et al.* (2004) found 46.9% availability of essential medicines in municipalities in Minas Gerais. Paniz *et al.* (2016) also observed that the reason for not obtaining 40% of the medicines needed to treat acute conditions in UBS in the South and Northeast regions of Brazil was unavailability in the SUS. This shows that the availability of medicines has been below the acceptable figure of 80% proposed by the World Health Organisation (WHO, 2009), compromising access to medicines for users of public health services in Brazil.

With regard to the infrastructure of pharmaceutical services, for example, Mendes *et al.* (2014) found that of 29,228 Basic Health Units that dispensed medicines, only 20% had a storage room and only 25% had a refrigerator for storing thermolabile medicines. Similarly, Vieira (2008) analysed data on pharmaceutical services in 597 municipalities and found inadequate storage conditions in 39% of them.

Among the assistance activities of pharmaceutical services, dispensing is the main activity, as it is carried out in every establishment that has medicines, and is a private act of the pharmacist (BRASIL, 1981). Dispensing is defined as the act through which one or more medicines are delivered to a user, in response to the presentation of a prescription drawn up by an authorised professional. At this point, it is assumed that the pharmacist will inform and guide the user on the appropriate use of the medicines (BRASIL, 1998). Often dispensing is the only time the user has contact with a pharmacist and it is also the last time the user has the opportunity to have contact with a health professional immediately before starting their treatment (MARIN *etal.*, 2003).

The practice of dispensing restricted to the act of supplying users with the medicines they require, without advocating pharmaceutical guidance and a more active stance by the professional in providing this service to the population, has been criticised for considering the pharmacist as a "medicine delivery person", to the detriment of the role of pharmaceutical care provider in the context of PS. Angonesi (2008) also emphasises that the practice of dispensing, defined as simply delivering medicines, reinforces the idea of the commercial nature of these products. Some studies have identified the inefficiency of the dispensing process carried out in this way (ARAÚJO *et al.*, 2008; ALENCAR *et al.*, 2011; SARTOR and FREITAS, 2014) and that this situation indicates the growing need for pharmacists to carry out more effective health promotion actions when dispensing. It is proposed that pharmacists develop skills in order to establish a relationship with the patient and turn the dispensing process into a procedure that guarantees quality care (GALATO *et al.*, 2008).

Given this situation, it can be concluded that users face many difficulties in obtaining their medicines at the right time and in the quantities needed for their treatment from primary care pharmaceutical services. It can also be seen that pharmaceutical services are still linked to the curative model, with the pharmacy serving medical demands and even with the advances in pharmaceutical services, with the definition and orientation of pharmaceutical services in Brazil, many problems jeopardise the objectives of guaranteeing access to medicines for the population and promoting rational use (ARAÚJO *et aL,* 2008; VIEIRA, 2010).

2.3 Access to medicines

Access to medicines is recognised by the United Nations as one of the indicators of progress in guaranteeing the right to health and the capacity of a health service to provide solutions (HOGERZEIL & MIRZA, 2011; HALAL *et aL,* 1994). It is an important concept in health policies, but it still doesn't have a precise definition, nor a closed evaluation model (LUIZA & BERMUDEZ, 2004; BIGDELI *et aL,* 2012), so much so that in Brazil and around the world, theoretical models vary in their definition of what access means and how this concept should be operationalised (WHO, 2000; OSCANOA, 2012; COSENDEY et aL, 2003; OSORIO-DE-CASTRO *et aL,* 2009).

According to the WHO (2000) and as presented by Luiza (2003), access to medicines is a construct made up of four dimensions:

- **Physical availability:** defined by the relationship between the type and quantity of products and services required and the type and quantity of services offered.
- **Geographical accessibility:** defined by the relationship between the location of products and services and the location of the eventual user of these products and services.
- **Suitability:** refers to the fit between the characteristics of products and services and the expectations and needs of users, as well as technical and legal operating standards.
- **Purchasing capacity:** defined by the relationship between the price of products or services and the user's ability to pay for them.

In addition to these, there is a cross-cutting dimension, which is also an essential component of access and cuts across all the previous dimensions, which is the Quality of Products and Services. Quality consists of applying medical science and technology in such a way as to maximise health benefits without increasing the risks. From the above, it is clear that access to medicines ultimately involves pharmaceutical services in order to guarantee the necessary quality, information on the rational use of medicines, sustainability and continuity of services (WHO, 2000; OSCANOA, 2012).

Considering that medication is one of the main health recovery strategies, it is necessary to carry out evaluations aimed at improving the population's access to medication (PANIZ, 2016). However, studies on access to medicines are generally divergent in terms of the concept used and how they measure and operationalise this concept (PENCHANSKY & THOMAS, 1981; LUIZA & BERMUDEZ, 2004; EMMERICK, 2011). A very common way of assessing access to medicines is through the availability dimension. In this sense, several authors translate obtaining medicines as access to medicines (BERTOLDI *et al.*, 2009; PANIZ *et al.*, 2010; WIRTZ *et al.*, 2008; BERAN et *al.*, 2016).

Despite the methodological differences, the results of studies focusing on availability have shown a similar panorama in relation to access to medicines by populations. A study that analysed access to medicines for chronic non-communicable diseases through interviews with 1867 individuals from five countries of different income levels (Uganda, Ghana, Kenya, the Philippines and Jordan) found prevalence rates of access ranging from 16.0% to 50.0% (VIALLE-VALENTIN *et al.*, 2015). In Brazil, Boing *et al.* (2013) found a prevalence of 45.8 per cent for obtaining prescription drugs. Tavares *et al.* (2016) also reported that, among adults and the elderly who had full access to treatment for chronic diseases in Brazil, only 47.5% had access free of charge.

CHAPTER 3

OBJECTIVES

3.1 General

To understand users' perceptions of access to medicines in pharmaceutical services in Divinópolis, Minas Gerais.

3.2 Specific

- To describe the profile of users of pharmaceutical services in primary health care in the municipality;

- To understand users' perceptions of access to medicines in pharmaceutical services;

- Characterising the dimensions of the concept of access to medicines based on the perceptions of users of pharmaceutical services

CHAPTER 4

METHODOLOGY

4.1 Context and Area

This work is part of the *"Servir Project: evaluating the role of pharmaceutical services in access to medicines in Divinópolis, Minas Gerais",* a qualitative study carried out in 2014 in Divinópolis. Divinópolis is considered the hub city of the Centre-West of Minas Gerais in the areas of health, commerce, education and industry and has a population of 213,016 inhabitants (IBGE, 2010).

In terms of health, the city is a macro-regional hub for 54 other municipalities, making it the headquarters of the Regional Health Management and a reference for medium and high complexity services, urgent and emergency care, oncological treatment, among others. The city is divided into health districts, five of which have pharmacies within the health units, with pharmaceutical services responsible for supplying the prescribed medicines to the population.

4.2 Project Serve

4.2.1 <u>Data collection and instrument</u>

The Servir Project data was collected between February and August 2014. In the case of users, semi-structured interviews were carried out in all five primary care pharmacy services in the municipality. Eligible users were individuals aged 18 or over, receiving medicines dispensed by the pharmacy at least six months before the interview and who agreed to take part in the study. In total, 186 users of PHC pharmaceutical services in Divinópolis were interviewed.

For data collection, guiding scripts were drawn up, based on the Guidelines for Structuring Pharmacies within the SUS (BRASIL, 2009), containing questions adapted from the literature (MACKEIGAN and LARSON, 1989; GOURLEY *et al,* 2001; LARSON et al, 2002; TRAVERSO et *al,* 2007) and questions developed by the research team. Questions related to pharmaceutical services were considered, ranging from aspects related to infrastructure to the service itself, as well as perceptions about access to prescribed medicines and the possible difficulties faced by users in gaining access to medicines at this level of care (LUZ *et al.,* 2013). Socio-demographic, economic and health-related information about the participants was also analysed. All the interviews were recorded and then transcribed.

4.2.2 Database construction

Thematic Content Analysis was carried out by the Servir Project research team using an iterative process (PATTON, 2015). To do this, the interviews were initially read independently and individually by the group members. Content and key terms were highlighted and copied from the transcripts into Microsoft Excel 2010 spreadsheets. A series of group analysis sessions then took place to develop the final coding structure of the highlighted themes. To establish the final coding structure, the "Coding Dictionary" was prepared, a reference document containing the concepts and definitions used in relation to each theme, which were based on three guidelines (WHO, 2000; STARFIELD, 1998; BRASIL, 2009).

4.2.3 Ethical issues

Ethical approval for the Servir Project was obtained from the Ethics Committee of the René Rachou Research Centre (Reference: 377.134). All participants signed an informed consent form. Anonymity and confidentiality were ensured and any identifying features such as the participant's name or location were removed to prevent participants from being identified.

4.3 Present Study

4.3.1 Data collection

For this investigation, interviews were selected from the Servir Project database until saturation occurred, i.e. when new themes no longer emerged from the interviews (PATTON, 2015). Sixty-nine interviews were selected and from these, quantitative socio-demographic, economic and health data was extracted (gender, age, marital status, schooling, monthly personal income and continuous use of medication). In addition, qualitative data was extracted on perceptions of physical space, comfort, waiting time and contact with the pharmacist; on obtaining medicines (obtaining all the medicines prescribed and the quantities obtained) and on dispensing practices (providing information on the name, indication, mode of use and possible adverse events of the medicines).

4.3. 2Data analysis

The data was quantified, i.e. variables were constructed from the qualitative data, the answers to which were transformed into categories. Numerical or ordinal values were assigned to the categories of the variables constructed. This procedure was adopted in order to make it easier to recognise patterns and make the information clearer (SANDELOWSKY *et al.*, 2009). A new database was then prepared using SPSS 22.0 software. The variables generated through this process were grouped into the dimensions of access to medicines "Physical Availability", "Adequacy" and "Quality", based on the concepts proposed in the WHO model, and were categorised as follows:

a) Physical availability

Table 1. Original variables, proposed variables and respective categorisations for the Physical Availability dimension

Original Variable	Variable New	Categorisation
Managed to get all the prescribed medication	Obtaining all medicines	(0) Yes (1) No
The quantities of medication received were sufficient for treatment	Obtaining sufficient quantities	(0) Yes (1) No

Source: Prepared by the author

b) Suitability

Table 2. Original variables, proposed variables and respective categorisations for the Suitability dimension

Original Variable	Variable New	Categorisation
Perception of the space in the dispensing area	Physical space	(0) Adequate (1) Fair (2) Inadequate
Perception of the comfort of the dispensing area	Comfort	(0) Comfortable (1) Fair (2) Uncomfortable
Perception of waiting time in the queue for service	Waiting time	(0) Adequate (1) Reasonable (2) Long/Very long

Source: Prepared by the author

c) Quality of service

Table 3. Original variables, proposed variables and respective categorisations for the Quality of services dimension

Original Variable	Variable New	Categorisation
Perception of contact with the pharmacist	Contacting a pharmacist	(0) Yes (1) No
Providing information on the name(s) and indication of the medicine(s)	Guidance on the name and indication of medicines	(0) Yes (1) No
Providing information on how medicines should be taken (timings/eating)	Instructions on the use of medicines	(0) Yes (1) No
Providing information about adverse events and what should be done if they occur	Instructions on possible adverse events	(0) Yes (1) No

Source: Prepared by the author

Descriptive statistics with the calculation of means, standard deviations, frequencies and proportions were carried out for all the new variables using SPSS 22.0 software.

CHAPTER 5

RESULTS

5.1 Sociodemographic, Economic and Health Profile

The analyses of the sixty-nine interviews showed that the group of participants was predominantly made up of female, elderly, married individuals with less than seven years of schooling and a monthly personal income of less than two minimum wages at the time of the study. The vast majority (92.4%) reported making continuous use of medication (Table 1).

Table 1. Characteristics of Users of Pharmaceutical Services. Servir Project, Divinópolis, 2014.

FEATURES	%
Female	63,8
Age	
20-39 years	13,6
40-59	40,9
>60	45,5
Mean (SD) (in years)	53,7 (±12,6)
Married [r]	60,9
Education	
< 7 years of study	62,3
Monthly personal income < 2 MW [r]	78,3
Uses medication continuously	
Yes	92,4

[2] marital status reported by the participants.
[·] Income expressed in minimum wages (MW), equivalent to R$ 724.00 at the time of the study.
Source: Prepared by the author

5.2 Users' perception of access to medicines

According to users' perceptions, three dimensions of the concept of access according to the WHO (2000) and Luiza (2003) were identified: availability, adequacy and quality of services. These dimensions and their respective variables are shown in the following tables.

5.2. 1Physical availability

The results of obtaining all the prescribed medicines and the quantities obtained are shown in Table 3.

Table 2. Physical availability as perceived by users. Servir Project, Divinópolis, 2014.

FEATURES	%
Obtaining all medicines	
Yes	47,8
No	52,2
Obtaining sufficient quantities	
Yes	69,8
No	30,2

Source: Prepared by the author

Less than half of the users reported having obtained all the prescribed medicines (47.8 per cent) and examples of the statements that generated these results are shown below:

"I couldn't get (all the prescribed medicines). *I either have to wait for them to arrive or buy them because I can't do without them, right?"* (USER 8)

"I needed metformin and I couldn't get it because it's out of stock, right? As the medicine comes from the government, it hasn't arrived at the pharmacy yet, that's what the guy told me. So there's no point in me staying here today!" (USER 39)

In addition, 30 per cent reported not being able to get enough medication for their treatment:

"There was one part missing. I think it was for 10 days." (USER 12)

"It came up short, so in that case I still have a bit at home... because usually we take it... sometimes we pass it on and it's left over." (USER 28)

<u>5.2. 2Adjustment</u>

The results regarding the adequacy of pharmaceutical services according to users can be seen in the table below:

Table 3. Adequacy related to pharmaceutical services, as perceived by users. Servir Project, Divinópolis, 2014.

FEATURES	%
Physical space	
Suitable	47,5
Reasonable	9,9
Inadequate	42,6
Comfort	
Comfortable	38,8
Reasonable	16,4
Uncomfortable	44,8
Waiting time	
Suitable	34,4
Reasonable	15,6
Very long/Long	50,0

Source: Prepared by the author

The majority of users rated the physical space of public pharmacies in Divinópolis as reasonable or inadequate (52.5 per cent):

"It's terrible. It's tight. There are times when the queue goes outside and it gets busy." (USER 6)

Regarding the comfort of the dispensing area, almost 45 per cent of users perceived it as uncomfortable:

"There are some benches there, but they're not comfortable. It should be more comfortable, have clean water, a toilet, right? There are a lot of elderly people who come, so they can get sick there, because they stand and the queue is very long, right?" (USER 9)

When asked about the waiting time from arriving at the pharmacy to being attended to, half of the interviewees considered it to be long or very long:

"That's a problem, right, it's too much here! We have to wait too long, too long. I think we need to improve that!" (USER 2)

5.2.3 Quality of Services

Users' perceptions of the quality of the pharmaceutical services offered can be seen in Table 4.

Table 4. Quality of pharmaceutical services as perceived by users. Servir Project, Divinópolis, 2014.

FEATURES	%
Contacting a pharmacist	
Yes	2,9
No	97,1
Name and indication of medicines	
Yes	9,1
No	90,9
Instructions on the use of medicines	
Yes	9,7
No	90,3
Instructions on possible adverse events	
Yes	4,5
No	95,5

Source: Prepared by the author

Almost all users (97.1 per cent) reported having no contact with a pharmacist when asked if they had ever looked for one in the pharmacies studied:

"No, I've never looked. I come here to get the medicine, you know, to get it... that's it! Except for that, we don't need to come, there's no need." (USER 6)

With regard to user guidance, three indicators were used to assess whether any information is passed on to users at the time of dispensing. Thus, 9 out of 10 users reported not receiving information on the name and indication of prescribed medicines, as well as instructions on how these products should be used:

"I already know the name, but he never said anything about these details (indication of medicines)." (USER 21)

"No, she didn't! (instructions on the use of medication) *It's routine stuff, right, if you go into too much detail it's going to get messy, so I think it's important that she delivers the medicine that's on the prescription and if she happens to see that the person has a headache, then it's an obligation, right?"* (USER 35)

Around 95 per cent of those interviewed also reported not receiving information about what should be done in the event of an adverse event:

"No, nobody says anything." (USER 40)

CHAPTER 6

DISCUSSION

Three dimensions of the concept of access emerged from analysing users' perceptions of access to medicines in the Pharmaceutical Services of Primary Health Care in Divinópolis: Physical availability, Adequacy and Quality of services.

The availability of medicines is often cited as a determining element in various studies on access to medicines and utilisation of health services (CHUKWUANI *et al.*, 2006, KIWANUKA et al., 2008; PARIYO *et al.*, 2009). It is also the dimension that has the strongest association with user satisfaction (AZEREDO *et al.*, 2009; MENDES *et al.*, 2012), despite the importance of all the other dimensions and the fact that the mere physical availability of products does not configure access to medicines (PANIZ, 2008).

Less than half of the users reported being able to obtain all the medicines prescribed, indicating a low physical availability of medicines in the services studied. In fact, several authors have pointed to the low availability of medicines in public pharmaceutical services (SILVA JÚNIOR & NUNES, 2012; BALDONI *et al.*, 2014). Considering that the continuous use of medicines observed in this study is common among adults and the elderly, the lack of medicines for daily use can lead to decompensation of users' chronic diseases (PANIZ, 2008).

The suitability of the products and services offered is related to the characteristics, needs and expectations of the user, as well as the suitability of the technical operating standards. In this sense, the results show that the services evaluated are at odds with the needs and expectations of the users taking part in the study, as well as being inadequate in relation to the guidelines and manuals that deal with the physical structure of pharmacies within the SUS.

According to the Ministry of Health Manual: Guidelines for structuring pharmacies within the SUS (BRASIL, 2009), it is essential that the internal and external areas of pharmacies are in good physical and structural condition, so as to allow hygiene for users and employees. It is also recommended that there be counters, tables and chairs in the dispensing area, allowing for greater interaction between the pharmacist and the user (BRASIL, 2009).

Users reported inadequate and uncomfortable physical space in the dispensing area of pharmacies, as well as long waiting times. Despite the lack of other similar studies to allow direct comparison of these findings, our results are in line with other authors. Bueno & Machado (2011) found an inadequate physical area, as well as problems with sanitising the premises, lighting and ventilation conditions in the public drug dispensing establishments they assessed. Cassara *et al.* (2016) also observed that the longer the waiting time in the queue, the lower the level of user satisfaction with pharmaceutical services.

Quality in health is the application of medical science and technology in a way that yields the maximum benefits for health without increasing its risks (DONABEDIAN, 1984). Thus, the quality of products and services is an essential dimension of access to medicines and one that cuts across all the others, since it is necessary to provide medicines, supplies and services with adequate characteristics in order to promote the correct use and ensure access to medicines in a qualified manner.

Users' perceptions were assessed in relation to the dispensing practices carried out in pharmaceutical services, since dispensing medicines is the central activity of these services and at this time users should be given guidance on the correct use of medicines, the importance of following the dosage and potential adverse events. All of these characteristics were used to assess dispensing practices and the data analysis showed that users do not usually receive information about medicines in the pharmaceutical services of the Divinópolis PHC.

The lack of information provided to users during dispensing in this case may be related to multiple factors, with two main ones standing out here. The first includes the poor structuring and organisation of pharmaceutical services, making the environment unsuitable for carrying out activities to guide and promote the rational use of medicines. Araújo *et al.* (2008) point out that in Basic Health Units, pharmacies generally occupy small spaces and are structured as a place to store medicines until they are delivered to the population. As such, the service usually takes place outdoors and with a lot of people around, which makes providing guidance to users in the pharmacy of the UBS practically impossible. Another important factor observed was that many of those interviewed were not aware of the importance of being advised about the medicines they use. It is therefore necessary to establish guidance activities on medicines for service users, since users' knowledge and understanding of pharmacotherapy, through guidance, are the most important variables for compliance with the prescribed drug treatment (TRÓCCOLI, 1990) and changing attitudes towards treatment depends, among other factors, on the information received by the user (CARVALHO *et al,* 1998).

The absence of information or misunderstanding of the instructions given by health professionals to patients can have consequences such as non-adherence to treatment, errors in the administration of medicines and an increase in the incidence of adverse effects, as well as other serious consequences that can worsen the patient's state of health (SILVA et *al.,* 2000; LAGE et a/., 2005). Therefore, the guidance on medicines provided to patients is fundamental to successful treatment, since the lack of it is one of the main causes of drug-related problems (MARIN et *al.,* 2003). In view of this, the quality of the services offered at the sites studied can be considered sub-optimal, which is in line with publications found in the literature (VIEIRA, 2007; ARRAIS *et al.,* 2007).

Overall, this study highlights important weaknesses in the pharmaceutical services of a major municipality in Minas Gerais and, given that the profile of the users studied is similar to that of Primary Health Care users in Brazil, as reported by other authors (AZIZ *et al.*, 2011; BALDONI *et al.*, 2014; BOING et al., 2013), the problems encountered can jeopardise regular access to medicines for continuous use, especially for the lower income population, where obtaining medicines free of charge is often the only way to get them (PANIZ, 2008).

The fact that the profile of users and the results found corroborate studies in the literature indicates that the methodological approach used in this study was well conducted and also made it possible to further explore the experiences and perceptions of the interviewees, satisfactorily describing the context studied. On the other hand, a limitation of this study is the use of secondary data, since the selection of variables in the database was pre-established according to the objectives of this research.

CHAPTER 7

CONCLUSION

Access to medicines in the pharmaceutical services of Primary Health Care in Divinópolis was considered deficient according to users' perceptions and the main dimensions of the concept of access to medicines that emerged were: physical availability, adequacy and quality of services. The emergence of these dimensions indicates that these were the critical points of the services according to the users' experiences and views.

Taken together, the results indicate the need for improvements in the municipality's Pharmaceutical Services in order to better structure the services and guarantee the provision of care to users. In this sense, there is also a latent need for user guidance practices to be established and, together, improvements to promote qualified access and the targeted use of medicines by the population.

REFERENCES

ACURCIO, F. A., organiser. **Medicines and Pharmaceutical Assistance.** Belo Horizonte: Coopmed; 2003.

ALENCAR, T.O.; BASTOS, V.P.; ALENCAR, B.R. *et al.* **Pharmaceutical dispensing: an analysis of legal concepts in relation to professional practice.** Rev Ciênc Farm Básica ApL 2011; 32(1): 89-94.

ANGONESI, D. **Pharmaceutical dispensing: an analysis of different concepts and models.** Cien Saude Colet. 2008; 13(Sup): 629-40.

ARAÚJO, A.L.A.; PEREIRA, L.R.L.; UETA, J.M. *et al.* **Profile of pharmaceutical care in primary care of the Unified Health System.** Ciência & Saúde Coletiva, 13(Sup):611-617, 2008.

ARRAIS, P.S.D.; BARRETO, M.L.; COELHO, H.L.L. **Aspects of the processes of prescribing and dispensing medicines in the perception of the patient: a** population-based study in Fortaleza, Ceará, Brazil. Cad Saude Publica 2007; 23(4):927-937.

AZEREDO, T.B.; OLIVEIRA, M.A.; LUIZA, V.L. etal. **User satisfaction with** pharmacy Services in the Brazilian National STD/AIDS Programme: validity and reliability issues. Cad Saude Publica 2009; 25(7): 1597-1609.

BALDONI, A.O.; DEWULF, N.L.S.; SANTOS, V. et al. **Difficulties of access to pharmaceutical services by the elderly.** Rev Ciênc Farm Básica ApL, 2014;35(4):615-621.

BERAN, D; EWEN, M.; LAING, R. **Constraints and challenges in access to insulin: a global perspective.** Lancet Diabetes EndocrinoL 2016; 3:275-85.

BERTOLDI, A.D; BARROS, A.J.; WAGNER, A. *et al.* **Medicine access and utilisation in a population covered by primary health care in Brazil.** Health Policy. 2009; 89(3):295-302.

BIGDELI, M.; JACOBS, B.; TOMSON, G. *et al.* **Access to medicines from a health System Perspective.** Health Policy and Planning. 28:692-704, 2012.

BOING, A. C.; BERTOLDI, A.D.; BOING, A.F. *et al.* **Access to medicines in the public sector: analysis of users of the Unified Health System in Brazil.** Cad Saude Publica. 2013; 29 (4): 691-701.

BRAZIL, Ministry of Health. 1997. **Basic Pharmacy:** 1997/98 Programme. Brasília: MS.

BRAZIL, Ministry of Health. **Assistência farmacêutica na atenção básica:** instruções técnicas para sua organização. 2. ed. Brasília : Ministério da Saúde, 2006b.

BRAZIL, Ministry of Health. **Guidelines for structuring pharmacies within the Unified Health System.** Brasília: Ministry of Health, 2009. 44 p.

BRAZIL, Ministry of Health. **Incentive for Basic Pharmaceutical Assistance:** what it is and how it works. Brasília: Ministry of Health; 2001.

BRAZIL, Ministry of Health. **Planejar é preciso:** uma proposta de método para aplicação à assistência farmacêutica. Brasília: Ministry of Health Publishing House, 2006a.

BRAZIL, Ministry of Health. **Ordinance GM/MS 204/2007.** Available at: < http://bvsms.saude.gov.br/bvs/saudelegis/gm/2007/prt0204_29_01_2007_co mp.html/bvs/saudelegis/gm/2007/prt0204_29_01_2007_comp.html > Accessed on: 20 May 2017.

BRAZIL, Ministry of Health. **Ordinance GM/MS n. 1.555, of 30 July 2013.** Provides for the financing and implementation of the Basic Component of Pharmaceutical Assistance within the scope of the Unified Health System (SUS). Available at:<http://www.saude.pr.gov.br/arquivos/File/0DAF/Portaria15552013CBAF.p dfpr.gov.br/arquivos/File/0DAF/Portaria15552013CBAF.pdf> Accessed on: 22

Dec. 2016.

BRAZIL, Ministry of Health. **Ordinance 176 of 8 March 1999.** Establishes criteria and requirements for the qualification of municipalities and states for the Basic Pharmaceutical Assistance incentive and defines amounts to be transferred. Available at:< http://bvsms.saude.gov.br/bvs/publicacoes/incentivo_assit_farm.pdf > Accessed on: 20 May 2017.

BRAZIL, Ministry of Health. **Pharmaceutical Services in Primary Health Care.** Brasília: Ministry of Health, 2014.

BRAZIL. National Health Council. **CNS Resolution 338/2004.** Available at:<portal.saude.gov.br/portal/arquivos/pdf/resol_cns338.pdf.> Accessed on: 24 Nov. 2016.

BRAZIL. National Council of Health Secretaries. **Pharmaceutical Assistance in the SUS.** Brasília: CONASS, 2007. 186 p.

BRAZIL. **Decree no. 68.806, of 25 June 1971.** Establishes the Medicines Centre (CEME). Federal Official Gazette, Brasília; 1971. Available at: <https://www.planalto.gov.br/ccivil_03/decreto/1970-1979/D68806.htm> Accessed on: 23 Nov. 2016.

BRASIL. **Decreto n. 85.878, de 7 de abril de 1981** .Estabelece normas para execução da Lei n° 3.820, de 11 de novembro de 1960, sobre o exercício da profissão farmacêutica, e dá outras providências. Diário Oficial da União, Brasília, DF, 9 April 1981. Available at: <http://www.planalto.gov.br/ccivil_03/decreto/Antigos/D85878.htm> Accessed on: 03 January 2017.

BRAZIL. **Law no. 8.080, of 19 September 1990.** Provides for the conditions for the promotion, protection and recovery of health, the organisation and operation of the corresponding services and makes other provisions. Federal Official Gazette 1990; 19 Sep.

BRAZIL. **Ordinance no. 3.916, of 30 October 1998.** Provides for the approval of the National Medicines Policy. Available at: <http//www.saude.gov.br/doc/portariagm3916/gm.htm> Accessed on: 24 Nov. 2016

BUENO, D. & MACHADO, A. **Avaliação dos dispensários do distrito sanitário Glória-Cruzeiro-Cristal Porto Alegre-RS.** Rev. APS 2011; 14(1):4-11.

CARVALHO, F.; JÚNIOR, R.T.; MACHADO, J.C.M.S. **An anthropological investigation into old age:** conceptions of arterial hypertension. Cad Saúde Pública 1998; 14:617-621.

CASSARO, K.O.S.; HERINGER, O.A.; FRONZA, M. etal. **Levei of satisfaction of clients of public pharmacies dispensing high-cost drugs in Espírito Santo, Brazil.** Brazilian J Pharm Sei 2016; 52(1): 95-103.

CHUKWUANI, C.M.; OLUGBOJI, A.; UGBENE, E. 2006. **Improving access to essential drugs for rural communities in Nigeria:** the Bamako initiative re-visited. Pharmacy World and Science 28: 91-5.

COSENDEY, M. A. E. **Análise de implantação do Farmácia Básica Programme:** um estudo multicêntrico em cinco estados do Brasil [thesis]. Rio de Janeiro: Sérgio Arouca National School of Public Health; 2000.

COSENDEY, M. A. E.; HARTZ, Z. M.; BERMUDEZ, J. A. Z. **Validation of a tool for assessing the quality of pharmaceutical Services.** Cadernos de Saúde Pública, Rio de Janeiro, v. 19, n. 2, p. 395-406, 2003.

DONABEDIAN, A. (1984). **The Quality of Medical Care:** Definition and Evaluation Methods. Mexico.

EMMERICK, I. C. M. **Dimensions and determinants of access to medicines in three Central American countries** [thesis]. Rio de Janeiro: Sérgio Arouca National Public Health Centre; 2011.

ENSOR, T. & COOPER, S. **Overcoming barriers to health service access: influencing the demand side.** Health Policy and Planning. 2004,19: 69-79.

GALATO, D.; ALANO, G.M.; TRAUTHMAN, S.C. et a/. **Dispensing medicines:** a reflection on the process for preventing, identifying and resolving problems related to pharmacotherapy. Revista Brasileira de Ciências Farmacêuticas, vol. 44, n. 3, juL/set, 2008.

GUERRA JR" A.A.; ACÚRCIO, F.A.; GOMES, C.A.P. *et al.* **Availability of essential medicines in two regions of Minas Gerais, Brazil.**Rev Panam Salud Publica. 2004; 15(3): 168-75.

HALAL, I.S.; SPARRENBERGER, F.; BERTONI, A.M. *et al.* **Evaluation of the quality of primary health care in an urban locality in the Southern Region of Brazil.** Rev Saúde Pública. 1994; 28:131-6.

HOGERZEIL, H. V. & MIRZA, Z. **The world medicines situation 2011:** access to essential medicines as part of the right to health. Geneva: World Health Organisation; 2011.

IBGE, Brazilian Institute of Geography and Statistics. **Cities: Minas Gerais - Divinópolis.** Available at:<http://cidades.ibge.gov.br/xtras/temas.php?lang=&codmun=312230&idtema=1& search=minas-gerais|divinopolis|censo-demografico-2010:-sinopse-> Accessed on: 14 Apr. 2017.

KIWANUKA, S.N.; EKIPARA, E.K.; PETERSON, S. *et al.* 2008. **Access to and utilisation of health Services for the poor in Uganda:** a systematic review of available evidence. Transactions of the Royal Society of Tropical Medicine and Hygiene 102: 1067-74.

LAGE, E.A.; FREITAS, M.I.F.; ACURCIO, F.A. **Information on medicines in the press: a contribution to rational use?** Cien Saude Colet 2005; 10(SupL): 133-139.

LUIZA, V.L. & BERMUDEZ, J.A.Z. Access to medicines: concepts and controversies. In: BERMUDEZ, J. A. S, OLIVEIRA, M.A, ESCHER, A. (org). **Acceso a medicamentos: derecho fundamental, papel del Estado.** Rio de Janeiro: Sérgio Arouca National School of Public Health, Oswaldo Cruz Foundation; 2004, p. 45-66.

LUIZA, V.L. **Access to essential medicines in Rio de Janeiro.** [Doctoral thesis] Rio de Janeiro; s.n; 2003. xiii, 227 p.

LUZ, T.C.B.; OSORIO-DE-CASTRO, C.G.S.; LUIZA, V.L. *et al.* **Projeto Servir: avaliação do papel de serviços farmacêuticos no acesso a medicamentos em Divinópolis, Minas Gerais.** Health and Environmental Education Laboratory (LAESA/CPqRR/Fiocruz/MG), 2013.

MARIN, N.; LUIZA, V.L.; OSORIO-DE-CASTRO, C.G.S. *et al.* **Pharmaceutical Assistance for Municipal Managers.** Rio de Janeiro: PAHO/WHO, 2003. 334p.

MENDES, A.C.G.; MIRANDA, G.M.D.; FIGUEIREDO, K.E.G. etal. **Accessibility to basic health services:** a road still to travel. Cien Saude Colet 2012; 17(11): 2903-2912.

MENDES, L. V.; CAMPOS, M.R.; CHAVES, G.C. *et al.* **Availability of medicines in basic health units and related factors: a cross-sectional approach.** Saúde em Debate, Rio de Janeiro, v. 38, n. especial, p. 109-123, 2014.

OLIVEIRA, L. C. F.; ASSIS, M. M. A.; BARBONI, A. R. **Assistência Farmacêutica no Sistema Único de Saúde:** da Política Nacional de Medicamentos à Atenção Básica à Saúde. Ciênc. saúde coletiva, Rio de Janeiro, v. 15, supl. 3, p. 3561-3567, 2010.

WHO. World Health Organisation. 2000. **Defining and Measuring Access to Essential Drugs, Vaccines, and Health Commodities.** Report of the WHO-MSH Consultative Meeting. Ferney-Voltaire, France: WHO-MSH.

WHO. World Health Organisation. 2009. **Implementing the third WHO Medicines Strategy 2008-2013.**

PAHO, Pan American Health Organisation/World Health Organisation. **Evaluation of pharmaceutical services in Brazil:** structure, process and results. Brasilia (Brazil); 2005.

PAHO, Pan American Health Organisation/World Health Organisation. **Pharmaceutical services based on primary health care.** PAHO/WHO Position Paper (La Renovación de la Atención Primaria de Salud en las Américas, n.6) PAHO, ed., Washington, DC: PAHO, 2013.

OSCANOA, T.J. **Access and usability to medications: a proposal for an operational definition.** Rev Peru Med Exp Salud Publica 29:119-26, 2012.

OSORIO-DE-CASTRO, C.G.S.; CHAVES, G.C.; RUIZ, A.M. *etal.* **A proposal for an evaluation model of pharmaceutical Services for malaria.** Cadernos de Saúde Pública, Rio de Janeiro, v. 25, n. 9, p. 2075-2082, 2009.

PANIZ, V.M.V.; CECHIN, I.C.C.F.; FASSA, A.G. *etal.* **Access to medicines for the treatment of acute conditions prescribed to adults in the South and Northeast regions of Brazil.** Cad. Saúde Pública, Rio de Janeiro, 32(4): 2016.

PANIZ, V.M.V.; FASSA, A.G.; FACCHINI, L.A. *et al.* **Access to continuous use medicines in adults and the elderly in the South and Northeast regions of Brazil.** Cad. Saúde Pública, Rio de Janeiro, v. 24, n. 2, p. 267-280, 2008.

PANIZ, V.M.V.; FASSA, A.G.; FACCHINI, L.A. *et al.* **Free access to hypertension and diabetes medicines among the elderly: a reality yet to be constructed. Cad.** Saúde Pública 26(6): 1163-1174: 2010.

PARIYO, G.W.; EKIPARA-KIRACHO, E.; OKUI, O. *et al.* 2009. **Changes in utilisation of health Services among poor and rural residents in Uganda:** are reforms benefitting the poor? International Journal for Equity in Health 8: 39.

PATTON, M. Q. **Qualitative Research & Evaluation Methods:** Integrating Theory and Practice. 4ª Edition. Saint Paul: SAGE Publications, Inc; 2015.

PEREIRA, N. C.; LUIZA, V. L.; CRUZ, M. M. **Pharmaceutical services in primary care in the municipality of Rio de Janeiro:** an evaluability study. Saúde debate, Rio de Janeiro, v. 39, n. 105, p. 451-468, 2015.

PEREIRA, N.C. **Monitoring the performance of pharmaceutical services in Primary Health Care:** seeking management qualification. 2013.124 f. Dissertation (Master's Degree) - Sérgio Arouca National School of Public Health, Rio de Janeiro, 2013.

PINHEIRO, R. M. **Serviços farmacêuticos na Atenção Primária à Saúde.**

Rev Tempus Actas de Saúde Coletiva, Brasília, DF, v. 4, n. 3, p. 15-22, 2010.

SARTOR, V. B. & FREITAS, S. F. T. **Model for the evaluation of drug-dispensing Services in primary health care.** Rev Saude Publica. 2014 Oct; 48(5): 827-36.

SILVA JÚNIOR, E. B.; NUNES, L. M. N. **Avaliação da assistência farmacêutica na atenção primária no município de Petrolina (PE).** Arquivos Brasileiros de Ciências da Saúde, São José do Rio Preto, v. 32, n. 2, p.65-69, 2012.

SILVA, T.; SCHENKEL, E.P.; MENGUE, S.S. **Level of information about medicines prescribed to outpatients at a university hospital.** Cad Saude Publica 2000; 16(2):449-455

STARFIELD, B. **Primary Care: Balancing Health Needs, Services, and Technology.** Revised Edition. Don Mills, ON: Oxford University Press; 1998.

TAVARES, N.U.L.; LUIZA, V.L. OLIVEIRA, M.A. *et al.* Free access to medicines for the treatment of chronic diseases in Brazil. Rev Saúde Pública. 2016; 50 (supl 2):7s.

TRÓCCOLI, B.T. **Obedience to medical prescriptions and disease control.** Medical Unit 1990; 15(2): 11-13.

VIALLE-VALENTIN, C.E.; SERUMAGA, B.; WAGNER, A.K. *et al.* **Evidence on access to medicines for chronic diseases from household surveys in five low- and middle-income countries.** Health Policy Plan. 2015; 30(8): 1044-52.

VIEIRA, F. S. **Pharmaceutical assistance in Brazil's public health system.** Rev Panam Salud Publica. 2010; 27(2): 149-56.

VIEIRA, F. S. **Qualification of pharmaceutical services in Brazil: inconclusive aspects of the Unified Health System agenda.** Rev Panam Salud Publica. 2008:24(2): 91-100.

VIEIRA, F.S. **Possibilities for pharmacists to contribute to health promotion.** Cien Saude Colet 2007; 12(1): 213-220.

WIRTZ, V.J.; REICH, M.R.; FLORES, R.L. *et al.* **Medicines in México, 1990-2004: systematic review of research on access and use.** Salud Publica Mex. 2008; S470-9.

ZULUAGA, G. C. R. **Pharmaceutical care and primary health care:** coordination, integrality and continuity of care in Pharmaceutical Dispensing and Care in Brazil. 2013. Dissertation (Master's in Public Health) - Oswaldo Cruz Foundation, Sérgio Arouca National School of Public Health, Rio de Janeiro, 2013.

ANNEX A

CONSOLIDATED OPINION OF THE CEP

RESEARCH PROJECT DATA

Research title: Servir Project: evaluation of the role of pharmaceutical services in access to medicines in Divinópolis, Minas Gerais.

Researcher: Tatiana Chama Borges Luz

Version 2

CAAE: 16094013.8.0000.5091

Proposing Institution: René Rachou Research Centre/ Oswaldo Cruz Foundation/ CPqRR/

Main Sponsor: René Rachou Research Centre/ Oswaldo Cruz Foundation/ CPqRR/ FIOCRUZ

OPINION DATA

Opinion number: 377.134

Reporting date: 26/08/2013

Project presentation:

Pharmaceutical services are part of the health services and carry out administrative, care and health education activities. Within the scope of the Unified Health System, these services must provide their users with access to essential medicines. However, despite the fact that promoting and expanding access to medicines for the population is one of the Brazilian government's commitments, problems still persist, resulting in a lack of comprehensive pharmaceutical care. Considering the difficulties faced by the population in accessing medicines, it is necessary to understand where the barriers are, which may lie in the provision of the supplies themselves, but may also be unrelated to the availability of the medicine. This project aims to evaluate the role of pharmaceutical services in access to medicines in a medium-sized municipality. It is a qualitative evaluation, analysing the content of official statements and texts. It is hoped to identify the constraints of management and health professionals with regard to access to medicines by the population, understanding the role and actions of the different actors in the process, including, in this sense, the pharmaceutical services.

users. This research should provide an opportunity to understand tensions in the political, social and economic fields and make it possible to anticipate management strategies for the health system. Data will be collected through interviews and focus groups.

Research Objective:

Primary objective: To evaluate the contribution of pharmaceutical services to access to medicines in Divinópolis.

Secondary objectives: To analyse the perception of users, managers and health professionals about pharmaceutical services with regard to access to medicines; To contrast the different perceptions of these actors and their consequence in relation to the effectiveness of access to essential medicines; To contrast the different perceptions of users with regard to access to medicines in public network pharmacies compared with the Popular Pharmacy of Brazil.

Evaluation of Risks and Benefits:
Risks: researcher says "not applicable".

Benefits: This research should provide an opportunity to formulate questions which, if better answered, could help to understand the lack of access to medicines, allowing for the design of more appropriate resolution strategies. In addition, with a view to anticipating management strategies for the health system, the study may make it possible to understand tensions in the political, social and economic fields. It is hoped that the results of this study can contribute to understanding access to medicines in the municipalities, thus supporting the formulation of local public programmes and policies, as well as new health technologies that take into account the specificities and needs of the population in the territories.

Comments and Considerations on the Research:
The research is relevant and could bring benefits to pharmaceutical care in the SUS. The recommendations suggested in the previous opinion have been met.

Considerations on the Terms of obligatory presentation:
The Terms of Presentation are now in accordance with the CEP standards.

Recommendations:
There isn't.

Conclusions or Pending Issues and List of Inadequacies:
I recommend that the project be approved by the CEP.

Opinion status:
Approved

Needs CONEP appraisal:

No

Final considerations at the discretion of the CEP:

After discussing the rapporteur's opinion, the Ethics Committee for Research Involving Human Beings of the René Rachou Research Centre/FIOCRUZ Minas decided to approve the project.

BELO HORIZONTE, 29 August 2013.

Signed by:
Naftale Katz
(Coordinator)

Address: Avenida Augusto de Lima, 1715

Neighbourhood: Barro Preto   **POSTCODE:** 30.190-002

UF: MG   **Municipality:** BELO HORIZONTE

Telephone: (31)3349-7825 **Fax:** (31)3349-7825 **E-mail:** cepsh-cpqrr@cpqrr.fiocruz.br

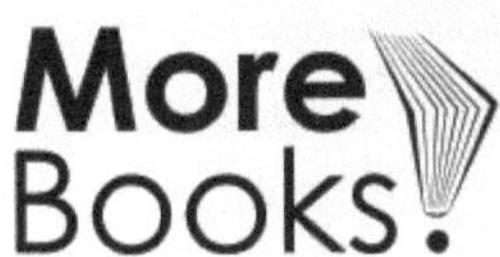

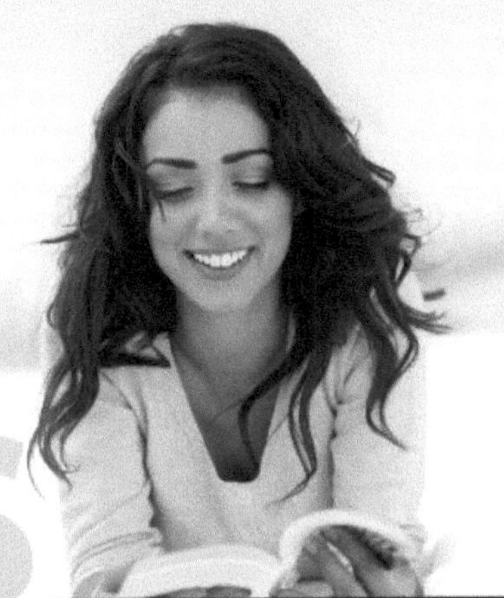

yes I want morebooks!

Buy your books fast and straightforward online - at one of world's fastest growing online book stores! Environmentally sound due to Print-on-Demand technologies.

Buy your books online at
www.morebooks.shop

Kaufen Sie Ihre Bücher schnell und unkompliziert online – auf einer der am schnellsten wachsenden Buchhandelsplattformen weltweit! Dank Print-On-Demand umwelt- und ressourcenschonend produziert.

Bücher schneller online kaufen
www.morebooks.shop

info@omniscriptum.com
www.omniscriptum.com

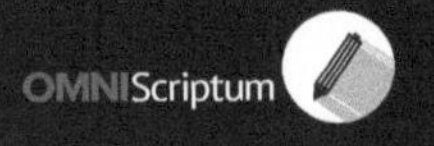

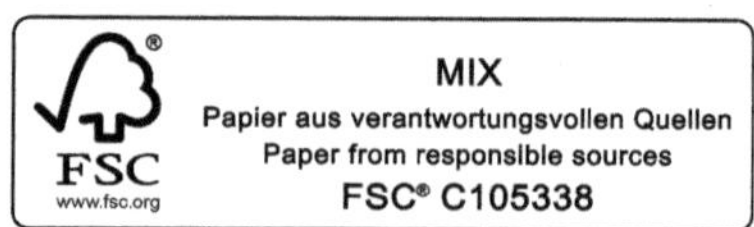

Printed by Books on Demand GmbH, Norderstedt / Germany